FALL IN LOVE WITH FITNESS

Guide for a Positive Relationship with Exercise

Fall in Love With Fitness

Photography: Lisa Lynn Photography & Design

Editorial: Sophie Elletson

Design: Dan Prescott-Bennett

The information provided in this book is for educational and informational purposes only and is not intended as medical advice. Always consult with a qualified health-care provider before beginning any exercise program, making changes to your diet, or implementing lifestyle modifications, especially if you are pregnant, nursing, have a medical condition, or are taking medication. The author is not responsible for any adverse effects or consequences resulting from the use of the information presented.

CONTENTS

Dedication

To my mom, Manette: For every mile you encouraged, every race you cheered, and every moment you made space for me to breathe. Thank you for not only believing in me, but also for watching the kids so I could chase this dream. You're no longer here to see it finished, but your love is laced into every page of this book.

To my husband and children: Thank you for cheering me on, asking how it's going, and reminding me every day why I love the miles I run, the words I write, and the life we're building together.

INTRODUCTION

I remember being pregnant with my first (full-term) child. I had already built a steady workout regimen, and working out made me feel like I wasn't pregnant. I would think, "Wow, I can't wait to get a jogging stroller and run with my baby!" I was committed to fitness beyond pregnancy. At the same time, I noticed how limited many people's thinking was. I was bombarded with comments like, "Just wait until you have that baby. You won't make it to the gym," or "Enjoy this now. You look great, but after having that baby, those days are over." The more I heard these comments, the more I felt this fire in me to prove them wrong. Why? Because I knew myself. Did I sometimes question it? YES. I wondered, "What is it that they know that I don't? Am I delusional?" But now, on the other side of those late nights, early mornings, and endless to-dos—and three BUSY athletic kids (ages eight, six, and three at the time of this book)—I'm here to tell you that YOU CAN do it.

This book isn't just for moms who struggle with a fitness routine. It's for every person who does. I keep being told to share my story to help others with fitness, so that is what I am here to do. I can't promise you'll find all the answers, and I don't even have them all, but I will share my journey and hope to offer a spark of encouragement.

You may be thinking, "Umm, I've heard this before. This isn't anything new." But the truth is, we all know what we are supposed to do, right? And it all seems simple enough. But somehow, it gets complicated. I hope I can help with that. Sometimes, hearing the message in a new way makes it click. Throughout this book, please think of me as your inner voice. On the one hand, I'm the voice that says, "Be easy on yourself, you're trying your best, give yourself some grace." Then there's that other voice that says, "You know you're capable of so much more. Let's see what happens if you do not quit this time." I believe in you, and I want you to believe in yourself as well. My curiosity about people's choices and my interest in helping others led me to get a degree in Psychology and then a Master's in Psychological Counseling, focusing on School Counseling in grades K-12. I believe we all have the power to change how we view our circumstances and that we have considerable control over our narrative. My counseling experience, my time as a health coach, and my genuine curiosity led me to bring this book to you. So please take what helps you, and leave or save the rest for later.

As you're reading, you'll find small reflections at the end of each chapter called "Your Next Move." These aren't meant to be lengthy assignments. They are gentle yet powerful prompts to help you turn inspiration into action. Think of them as small action steps to remind you that growth does not happen all at once. Everything begins with one decision and one new habit at a time.

So, are you ready? Great. But before you continue reading, promise yourself one thing: you won't quit this time.

CHAPTER 1.
A TRIP DOWN MEMORY LANE

Let's start from the beginning, back to little me, rather than my first pregnancy, because fitness had already been part of my life before then. However, before I take you back, I want to share some research. An article by USC about student-athletes found that many struggle to make fitness part of their lives after the school sports are over, which makes sense because now it is solely up to them to make it happen. In a Harvard poll, 3 in 4 children play sports, but only 1 in 4 of those children become adults who continue to play. Among parents, just 28% of mothers get the recommended daily exercise. These numbers highlight that there is much room for improvement when it comes to lifelong fitness. But don't be discouraged; many factors can disrupt one's commitment and discipline around fitness.

So, whether you've never lifted a weight or stepped into a gym, or you ran track as a teenager, neither path guarantees lifelong fitness. Both situations can be intimidating. I have had several conversations with former student-athletes who felt lost when they no longer had their structured sports and the direction of their coaches and/or parents regarding fitness and health. We all have different paths, and it's important to recognize and honor your unique journey. Everything, including your decision to pick up this book, has led you right up to this moment.

Back to my formative years. As a 90s kid, I played outside constantly with my older brother (and later, my younger sisters and younger brother), going home for a quick midday sandwich, then back out again until the streetlights came on. I don't recall my parents pushing sports, but my dad took us to the park almost every weekend to ride bikes, play soccer, and run around. We were active. I also have vague memories of watching my dad always doing some stretches and jumping jacks when he woke up each morning before starting his day. He loved watching soccer and boxing, and still does. My mother walked a lot with us, as she didn't get a driving license until I was a little bit older. I also remember dancing with her, which was always fun.

I loved playing with my older brother in the streets of the many neighborhoods we moved to, Brooklyn, Queens, Long Island. We played everything, from basketball to football, including racing each other down the block. But it never crossed my mind to play official sports. I thought they were something famous professionals did. That changed when I was in the 6th grade. I had just moved to Long Island from Queens and felt like I didn't belong there; there were not many people who looked like me. But in gym one day, we all had to try something called rotary track. I don't know if I would have otherwise. Each student had to race each other, and the fastest would be chosen to participate in a track meet at the High School. This meet would include my town's fastest kids from each grade and elementary school. I was chosen for the 55-meter race. I don't remember where I came in the race, but I remember how I felt: nerves before, yet elation after. Those emotions will never leave me.

Before racing, I was so nervous that I was shaking and sweating. My heart was beating so fast. The high school track where it took place felt so big, even though it was the same size as the track we practiced on in gym class. I felt as if I did not belong there—classic impostor syndrome. After the race though, everything changed. I remember thinking, "This feels good. I have to do this again. I need to do this again." So, when I entered middle school later that year, I joined the track team. To my pleasant surprise, the coach, Ms. Barnes, was also the English teacher. I admired her so much. In a predominantly White town in the year 2000, I remember how happy I was to have a Black woman as a teacher because I didn't feel so alienated. She was inspiring and taught all of us to try our best, believe in ourselves, and never forget to "run pretty." She was and still is a force.

My mother never understood my fascination with the sport; she was baffled by my running obsession. Nevertheless, she supported me because she saw how happy it made me, and she was genuinely one of my biggest supporters. And because of Coach Barnes, I knew that running would be a part of my life for a long time. Running fueled me. It made me feel as if nothing else in life mattered. If I was having a bad day, running after school would be there to save me. At the same time, I connected with friends who felt like sisters too. We always complained during practice, of course. But what kept me coming back was how I felt after practice and after track meets. With that, I decided without thinking twice to run in high school.

High school track presented new challenges. At first, I struggled with wanting to quit but also wanting to prove myself as a freshman. Being 14 among other older runners felt intimidating and too serious for a bubbly person like me. We ran six days a week, which meant I spent my Saturday mornings doing that instead of watching cartoons in my pajamas with my siblings. We also lifted weights and did a lot of core work. It was intense. We ran in the rain, we ran in the snow, we ran in hail, the heat, and the cold. Looking back, I can see that these tough conditions shaped me as an athlete and a person. I started questioning if I had what it took to be a runner. But my high school coach, Coach Schaefer, taught me that my self-doubt, fear, and anxiety were not reasons for me to quit; they were all reasons for me to continue. He was an amazing and wise human being. He taught me that these emotions were because I cared about the sport and wanted to do well. I still remember his advice today, especially during new challenges, such as college track.

I should say here that I promise this book is not about running; everything will eventually connect!

In college, I again seriously questioned my abilities. After four years of high school track, being in a new environment, with classes, making new friends, and different teams, was a lot for me to process. I only ran for one semester in college, but that one semester changed my life. Quitting the team was one of the toughest decisions, but it wasn't because I'd fallen out of love with running. Looking back, I made that decision because it was nothing like high school track, and I had so much more to juggle. I was a sprinter and hurdler, but the team mainly consisted of distance runners. I didn't feel I would flourish on the team and I feared my talents would go to waste. So, I quit. Ironically, I embraced distance running later.

After quitting the team, something that had been so consistent in my life from age 12 to 18, during the forming of my adolescence, was now gone. A friend I had recently made, Carolyn, who also loved running and ran in high school, helped me navigate this difficult time. We started running 3 miles together almost daily before class. It wasn't easy, and she often had to stop for me to catch my breath, especially after a big hill that we always ran up. We called the route "The Head Honcho." She was fit and so patient. She filled me up with affirmations and encouraged me every step of the way. This was when I started understanding the value of health and fitness. Not having a team anymore made me realize how impactful running had been on my mental health and overall mood.

Movement became my personal outlet. It wasn't about transformation or proving anything; it was simply how I cleared my head and reconnected with myself. I was building something that would serve me in the hardest seasons ahead: consistency, patience, and self-trust. Those lessons would meet me again when motherhood entered the picture.

When you read this chapter, I want you to realize that nothing happened overnight. It was a process. I went from not knowing I could even run fast as a 6th grader to becoming a distance runner. But I faced many hurdles along the way. I kept letting my negative thoughts dictate what I thought I could do, which I will delve into later. I need you to remember this and repeat it to yourself multiple times when you are on your journey and figuring everything out. When you try to make a change too quickly, it rarely lasts. The initial momentum runs out. However, when you are patient, give yourself room to make missteps and grow; that is when you will flourish.

When I found out I had high cholesterol in high school, for example, I cut out fast food entirely for a few weeks. Being a young athlete, I didn't always make the healthiest choices. Given that my family has some health issues already, such as high blood pressure, I started to get a little nervous about the path I had been on. I felt great, and my cholesterol did go back to normal. But then, I started going back to those drive-throughs. The change was temporary, and my habits instantly returned to where they were before. It is often when we try to suddenly change our habits that we fail at our goal. I realized I had to gradually cut down. As I made healthier choices, my body started to reject unhealthy ones.

I remember the day I knew it really was time to change my fast-food habit. I was on my way to work and didn't have time to make breakfast, so I got a meal at a very popular place. By the time I took the 20-minute ride to work, I started feeling extremely sick. I ran to the bathroom, and it was not pretty. However, it was only after I had my second child in 2017 that I stopped eating there completely. My journey was a roller-coaster, but I finally got there!

Similar to your fitness journey, you will not have a linear route. But then your body will signal to you when it needs you to do something. When your body speaks, it is crucial to listen. I know that if I skip being active for more than two days or if I have days of not eating the foods that I know will properly fuel my body, my physical and mental health will indeed suffer. You want to reach that point where the discipline kicks in and keeps you going on days you think you cannot.

Once the discipline kicks in, it takes a lot to take you away from your goals. You may find yourself doing things that you never thought you would. I went from quitting a college track team that focused on distance running to completing so many distances I said I would never even attempt. I even trained for a full marathon twice while juggling my three children. Start by building discipline because those things that once seemed impossible will slowly start to shapeshift into "maybe one day."

Your Next Move: Recall your earliest positive memory of movement. It can be a sport, a dance, a run. Jot it down in your phone or journal so you can revisit it when motivation fades.

CHAPTER 2.
THE POWER OF HEALTH

Before having children, I worked out whenever and for as long as I wanted. While I had to fit it in between work and school, it was much easier with only myself to consider.

When I became pregnant in December 2013, I had no idea that the following events would escalate my fitness journey. I knew I was pregnant pretty quickly. I took a test on New Year's Eve, and it was negative. But I knew it had to be wrong because I had never been this tired in my entire life. Not even with staying up late writing school papers. I took another test on January 1, 2014, and it was positive. I was elated. When I called my doctor, my first question was whether I could continue working out, and he said yes. I kept up with my runs and gym trips, keeping my heart rate low and feeling proud. Then, we went to the doctor. Even though I was only six weeks along, I saw hopeful concern on the ultrasound tech's face as she told us that the heartbeat wasn't steady and was flickering in and out. But she assured us that the flicker in the heartbeat was probably due to how early it was in the pregnancy. Naturally, when we returned at 10 weeks, we hoped to see and hear a strong heartbeat.

I remember that day very clearly. My husband and I went into the office cautiously optimistic. The tech, who had been very chatty and happy, took a look at the screen and became quiet and focused. Soon after, her face changed. She said, "I'll be right back." Not knowing that the tech wasn't supposed to say anything, I immediately asked, "Is everything okay??" She repeated that she would be right back. One of the doctors in the office walked in a few moments later and told us that she was very sorry, but there was no heartbeat, and the next step would be to schedule a D&C. I couldn't come to terms with it. Even up until the day of the procedure, I wanted them to do an ultrasound to double-check. Even with my HCG levels (the pregnancy hormone that doctors track to confirm growth) dropping, I thought maybe they would rise again.

On the morning of the procedure, I bled at the hospital before going into surgery. It was February 14, 2014. The blood was a slight relief because it made me realize that things probably wouldn't have worked out. They did an ultrasound to be sure, but there was still no heartbeat. I was an absolute emotional wreck after the D&C. Yet, this was the true start of my health journey, and I never looked back.

Healing isn't linear. Even after deciding to exercise again, I still found myself waiting, wondering, and hoping each month for a different outcome. I am very well aware that many people deal with infertility, and a few unsuccessful tries did not mean that I would not ever get pregnant. But that didn't help me in the months that followed my miscarriage. Month after month, my pregnancy tests came up negative. I remember crying on the bathroom floor so hard that my whole body ached. I was starting to get depressed and feel lost. I went from taking comfort in talking to my husband about it to just feeling angry. Not toward him, but just everything. My husband handled it way better than I did, on the outside, anyway.

Having a degree in psychology and counseling, I knew I couldn't continue like this. I was losing myself and lashing out at my husband. I did not yet know what my plan was, but I knew I needed one. I decided one day to channel all these feelings into running and changing my diet as much as possible while still enjoying the things I loved. I like to call myself The Research Queen. I research anything I am going through until I cannot research it anymore. I found that my chances of getting pregnant would be better if I took very good care of myself, so I wanted to control anything that I could. Even though my doctor reassured me how common miscarriages were, I couldn't help but blame myself from time to time. So, I did what any sane person would: I signed up to run the Long Island Half Marathon. I had never run 13.1 miles and had no idea how to complete this task. I just knew that I needed something that would make me feel like I was in motion again. My husband was already farther along in his running journey, and I thought it would be a fail-proof plan to challenge myself and train for a half-marathon, especially since he would be running as well. Training helped me cope. With each passing week, I ran farther than ever and started feeling very hopeful. I told myself that I would stop worrying about getting pregnant, enjoy my husband, and focus on my health and goals. I wanted to ensure that I was in the best shape of my life for when I would be blessed with pregnancy again.

I started to realize that running wasn't just about moving forward physically. It became a way of learning to breathe again and regaining trust in myself. After spending so much time feeling so disconnected from my body, running helped bridge the gap. It reminded me that my body wasn't broken; it was healing and adapting. I was finding strength in places I didn't know existed.

By the time the race came, I wasn't just running for the finish line anymore. I was running for every version of myself that had felt lost, uncertain, or small. On the day of the half-marathon, my husband ran every mile with me, and we finished together holding hands. During my next cycle, just a month later, I got pregnant. I remember running to our bedroom that morning I saw the positive on the test and shaking my husband out of his sleep. Let's just say I think I scared him a little with how I woke him up. Seeing that positive pregnancy test felt like a full circle moment because I knew that during the waiting period, I had done my part to care for myself. That experience taught me that health is not just about effort but also a partnership with your body. My body and I had been through something heavy, and instead of giving up on it, I decided to believe in it again. Adopting that mindset shift changed everything. I no longer worked out just to control the outcome. I moved out of gratitude, I ate to nourish, and I rested without guilt.

This time around with pregnancy, I was cautious with my workouts just in case because my anxiety was heightened. I did start to feel less anxious around week 14, and as the pregnancy progressed and I was able to feel my baby throughout the day. I saw why the naysayers I mentioned in the intro said I probably wouldn't be able to work out. This pregnancy was so very different. I knew it would go to term or at least make it further because of how strong I felt the symptoms from the very beginning. I was nauseous all day. Working out was the only thing that gave me relief, but then the nausea would return and last until around 9:00 PM each night. I had very intense headaches that made my mornings extremely slow, and I was even more exhausted than before. But still, I somehow pushed through.

Many people didn't understand why I didn't just rest instead of working out. I tried to explain to them the benefits of working out during pregnancy and how it made me feel in the moment and for a little bit after. In my experience with all three babies, I didn't feel pregnant when I worked out. I felt unstoppable. That is what kept me going. I kept my doctor involved, and he always pushed me to keep going.

Working out during pregnancy is widely accepted now, but even back in 2014, I faced a lot of backlash from gymgoers. I was signed up at an all-women's gym at the time, and many elderly women would say offensive things to me, like, "You're going to kill that baby." I sense now that these are probably the same women who would say something like, "Working out as a mom is selfish." Every time I walked into the gym, they all stared at me with major disdain.

I think we all know now that it isn't selfish to work out. Working out during pregnancy helped me start my parenting journey with the discipline I would need to get in workouts between feedings, fatigue, life, and marriage. Would it have been perfectly fine if I chose not to work out during my pregnancy? Sure. But I will tell you that I worked out until the very end of all three of my pregnancies, which is one of the things I am most proud of. I am not a doctor, but our pediatrician mentioned that staying active during pregnancy may have played a role in our kids' early physical development (strength, coordination, motor skills).

Working out is not selfish. It is something you're doing for your future baby (if you want to have kids) and yourself. Whether you're walking, doing yoga, or going for walks, if cleared to do so by your physician, the benefits are there. Looking back, that season was the foundation for everything I believe about fitness now. It showed me that health is not just a number or a goal on paper. It's the power to rebuild when life falls apart, even when motivation is absent. It is the power to nurture your body through all types of seasons.

Health and fitness gave me something I did not know I was missing. Trust. It helped me trust that I could start again and go further than I ever believed, even if I didn't think I was ready. It helped me to trust that small steps over time would lead to something bigger and unshakable. That's what I want every reader to know. You do not have to have it all figured out to begin your own health journey. You just have to start truly caring for yourself in the middle of it all.

Your Next Move: Choose one small act of care today. Go for a walk, drink more water, cook yourself a real meal. Then, keep doing it and build consistency.

CHAPTER 3.
FITNESS IS A CHOICE, RIGHT?

Fitness is a choice. I believe it, I feel it, breathe it, and live it. But I also know that if certain things aren't in place, it doesn't matter how much you want to be fit; it won't happen, especially as a busy parent with busy children. I learned that pretty quickly. But before I continue, I am also well aware that there are people who have limitations or chronic illnesses that may prevent them from engaging in certain physical activities. For some, movement looks different, and that's okay. Health is not one-size-fits-all. It's not always about miles or weights or high intensity. Sometimes, it's about breathing through pain, honoring where your body is today, or doing what you can with the energy you have.

I want to acknowledge that for anyone reading this who's navigating illness, fatigue, or recovery, your effort still counts. You are still doing the work. You're showing up in ways the world may never see, and that matters. Fitness doesn't have to mean doing everything. It means doing what you can, consistently, and with love for your body.

For me, just doing what I can became especially clear after having my first child. When she was almost one, I started training for another half-marathon. After training for and running that race on barely any sleep, I realized I had to make some significant changes. I kept thinking, "Her sleep will get better." But my daughter was 1 year and 2 months old when I ran that race, and her sleep was getting progressively worse. So, I did my research. I realized that I was unintentionally teaching her to wake up at certain times or providing crutches for her to fall asleep.

Listen, some people have no problem sleeping with their kids in their beds or rocking them to sleep for a while, if not forever. These methods, though, would not fit what we wanted for our family, and it honestly wasn't helping her or us get the best sleep. So, my husband and I hesitantly agreed that we would sleep-train her. Sleep is a learned skill. This is a tricky and touchy topic, and some parents disagree. I disagreed at first too, before I truly understood. For those interested, there are gentle methods that don't involve letting your baby cry for hours. Sleep training is not usually recommended if your child has colic or has special needs.

It was HARD. But it was a few days of hard traded in for a lifetime of excellent sleep. I won't go into the details about the actual sleep training methods, as every family has different needs. But I will say that I used to think my daughter was just an "unhappy baby." She was grumpy a lot of the time. After sleep training her, I felt so guilty because she woke up happy and smiling after her first night of uninterrupted sleep! My poor girl was just exhausted. After making it to the other side of sleep training, I knew what timeframe she would sleep at night and when she would wake up in the morning. I could work out before she woke up in the mornings, and at night, my husband and I could have date nights. It was an entirely different and well-rested life. So, when we had our second baby, I made sure not to do certain things I had done before, such as waiting too long to put him down after he fell asleep in my arms after nursing. He actually didn't need much sleep training, probably because, as a mom of two, I wasn't able to get to him as quickly as I could when it was just my daughter. He learned to settle on his own sometimes. By 9 months old, I realized he was ready, and he didn't even cry the first time I let him put himself to sleep. If you look at some foundations of sleep training, one important factor is not to always rush in the second your baby cries, as sometimes, they're just crying in their sleep and can settle back on their own. Our second child also was accustomed to hearing the everyday sounds around the house and became a deeper sleeper than our daughter, who experienced a lot of quiet as a baby.

Our third baby, who was exclusively breastfed for two years, showed signs of being ready to sleep independently at five and a half months. I struggled more with the third baby internally because he did not take bottles or pacifiers, although we tried everything, and would wake up at night looking for me every hour (before sleep training). I was in new territory, but I had learned that the little things I did from the beginning would help the whole process go easier. With him, I already knew that if I waited the magical 5 minutes, he would most likely settle and fall asleep whenever he would cry out in the night. There are certain ages for these milestones. Please realize that even after the newborn phase, in my opinion and experience, babies need extra connection even for some months after, depending on the baby. I learned pretty quickly with each kid what a cry or a sound meant that they needed.

What matters most is that you and your partner are on the same page and ready to be consistent. Inconsistency in sleep training confuses a child. Many parents will go into sleep training excited and determined, only to quit one or two days in, which now puts them in a worse spot than before. And honestly, this is like working out. You cannot go into something and quit once it gets tricky. You have to keep going to see what happens on the other side. However, everyone knows their child best. You have to discern whether you're giving up on the sleep methods for yourself or your child. And also, there were nights when I put my own spin on the technique because we know our children. For example, one method I tried was one where I sat in the room, and every third night, I moved further away from the bed, reassuring my baby with my voice. This was harder for them. My kids preferred me out of the room and out of sight, with an occasional voice through the monitor or behind the door telling them that I am still near and I love them.

I include this hot topic of sleep training because whenever I talk to parents who say they don't have the time or energy to focus on their fitness, it usually starts with their sleep and their child(ren's) sleep. Doing anything else in life is impossible if your sleep is out of whack. Whether you have children or not, it starts with your sleep.

Once your sleep is under control, it will be easier to know when you will work out, and your eating habits and stress levels will be more regulated. But what happens if everyone sleeps well now, but you still don't feel like it? Re-read the title of this chapter. It is your choice what you end up doing. No one will push you out of that bed and make you do it but yourself. Although I've definitely had my husband nudge me before after my alarm went off to get a training run done.

With my background in psychology, I know that other factors besides sleep can stand in the way of choosing to work out. Much of this journey is mental. In fact, most of it is. There are so many reasons people develop an antagonistic relationship with fitness. Sometimes it's rooted in fear, comparison, or self-doubt. For years, I told myself I wasn't built to be a distance runner. I really thought that it could never be me. I put myself in a box and stayed there, convincing myself I couldn't go further. I wish I had realized sooner that those limits weren't real; they were just stories I kept repeating to myself.

Mental toughness is often overlooked, but it's one of the most powerful skills you can build. You're already showing signs of it simply by picking up this book. It means something inside you wants to change, and that part of you deserves your full attention. While I'm not focusing solely on mindset here (there are amazing books and podcasts that do), I do want to remind you to check in with yourself mentally. Ask yourself if the only thing holding you back is the belief that you can't. Because if that's the case, I promise, you can and you will.

But there's another layer we need to talk about, and that's mental health. There's a difference between needing motivation and managing something deeper. I've worked with people walking through depression, anxiety, infertility, body dysmorphia, and more. If you're carrying something heavy like that, please don't punish yourself for what you haven't been able to do. Healing takes time, and your path may look different from someone else's. The goal isn't perfection; it's patience. Work with a therapist or doctor you trust, and take care of your mental wellbeing the same way you would care for your physical body.

Because even during those seasons, there's still a choice. Maybe the choice is not about how fast you can move, but about how gently you treat yourself while you move through it. Some people choose to stay in the "why me?" space, and others find a way to rise above it, one (sometimes very slow) step at a time. Wherever you are, your choice still matters.

The beautiful thing about realizing that you do have a choice is that it changes everything. You start to fall in love with the process—not just the workouts, but the energy, the peace, the confidence that follows. You realize that fitness is bigger than the physical; it's a mirror for life. When you show up for your body, you remind yourself that you can also show up for everything else. It won't always be seamless, but it will definitely be worth it.

Your Next Move: For the next 24 hours, pay attention to the choices you make that impact your health. Capture one in your notes app or journal as proof that you're in control.

CHAPTER 4.
PREPARE WELL OR FAIL

Preparation is one of those things we know we should do. We've heard it from parents, teachers, coaches, and motivational speakers. Yet somehow, many of us still avoid it. Maybe it feels tedious, or maybe it just requires slowing down when we'd rather keep going. Often, it comes down to instant gratification. Preparing for the next day the night before means saying no to what feels good right now in exchange for something that won't pay off until tomorrow, or even further down the road.

I grew up with Caribbean immigrant parents who truly instilled the importance of structure. As a kid, I despised it. Why did I have to pick out my clothes for the next day of school and iron them? My older brother had this routine down perfectly. Hearing it from him hit differently than hearing it from my parents because kids are stubborn, right? He would choose his outfits for the entire week, down to which sneakers he'd wear each day.

He taught me that doing this made mornings smoother and helped me start the day feeling confident. And honestly, he was right. I know that when I pick an outfit in my head, and it doesn't look how I imagined, I end up frazzled, wasting time trying to find something that feels good. What I didn't realize back then was that this same principle would later apply to the success or failure of my workouts.

Fast forward to adulthood—work, college, grad school, and now my fitness life— and that lesson has stayed with me. I still pick out my clothes ahead of time because it removes one more excuse to procrastinate. Preparation isn't glamorous, but it always pays off.

When you have to make more decisions in the morning (or any time you choose to work out), there is a considerable chance that you will be hindered. You might get distracted and start doing something else or forget about it altogether. Also, just thinking about what you need is not the same as actually getting it together. I say this because I have done this, and sometimes it works out great, but other times, it doesn't. Especially if it's early morning and I'm trying to be quiet as I get my things together.

I choose every single thing that I need for my workout. This includes but is not limited to my outfit, bra, underwear, socks, scrunchies for my hair, hat, energy drink, water, weights, you get the picture. I also know what I will eat before beginning, which workout I am doing, and how long it will take. So, the only thing I have to do really is get myself out of bed and into the bathroom, and then I go on autopilot. I even take it a step further to know which podcast or audiobook I'll be listening to before my workout even begins. I set my phone alarm to a song that will wake me up in a good mood and then go to bed knowing I am prepared for the upcoming day. Before having children, you may be able to get away with less preparation. But if you already struggle with pushing yourself to get your fitness in check, any excuse to skip it or save it for later will hinder your success.

Let's be realistic here: sometimes I choose to relax instead of completing all these tasks, especially if it was a late night with kids' sports. But I also attempt to do this much earlier in the day if necessary. The idea is to prepare as much as you can. My kids are getting older now and have their choice of clothes sometimes, so either they or I choose their clothes for school the next day. Along with that, I get their clothes ready for their after-school sports. I even take it a step further and choose their pajamas for when they come home and take a bath/shower. I know this seems like a lot and feels like a lot. You eventually get into a rhythm and groove though, and the kids start to help.

They will wake up in the morning and already choose their pajamas for that night. The great thing about this too is that they are watching and getting a front-row view of discipline and preparation.

Something that can really take time in the morning, if not completed the night before, are school lunches, snacks, and water. Granted, if you're waking up early for a workout, you may have more time, but you still never know what a morning may present you with. There have been many times while working out that a kid woke up a little earlier than usual because they have a nosebleed, a bad dream, or they just miss mommy and daddy. They are human after all, and as much as we can try to predict sleep and wake times, things will always happen. Those interruptions can skew the whole morning. So, something else we do when we get the calendar for school lunches, is that the kids look at the calendar and they either tell me or write their names on the days they plan on eating the school food and which days they want food from home. So then I know what to do to prep for their lunch and snacks.

I'd like to take a pause here and say that this may sound as if I figured it out on the first try. I did not. This has been and still is trial and error. Even though my eldest is now 10, I still feel very new to motherhood in many ways. Every time one of my children enters a new phase, I feel like I'm starting over right alongside them. I want you to know that we're all figuring this out together. My hope is that the things that have worked for me will either help you directly or inspire you to find your own rhythm. Mornings will always have some chaos because that's just real life. But preparation helps you keep it from becoming overwhelming. Don't make it harder on yourself by adding more to your plate than necessary.

I would also like to add that no matter the time that I am working out, I am prepared. When my babies were babies, most of my workouts happened at night after breastfeeding them so that I was 1. empty and they were 2. fed and happy. It was also easier knowing that my husband was home and ready to step in if they woke up during a workout. So, even if you are working out at 9:00 PM, it still helps to know what you will be eating and wearing. And if the workout is happening at nap time or after school drop-off, it helps if you are already dressed for the workout to prevent you going back on your word. I will admit that after years of doing all of this, it does get easier to still complete a workout if I didn't prepare perfectly, but even so, it is still a hurdle that I do not always want to jump over.

At first, doing all this preparation will seem tedious. Some days will be better than others. But then you'll start to experience all the benefits, and I challenge you to use those feelings when you simply don't feel like doing a workout. Start to see your workouts as a normal and natural part of your day. I mean, you wouldn't go to work unprepared for a presentation, would you? That would be horrifying. Your workouts should uphold the same standards because letting yourself down should also be horrifying. This may sound a little dramatic. However, the way you show up for yourself first and foremost sets the tone for other situations and relationships in your life. Do not underestimate the power of preparation.

Your Next Move: Prep one thing today that will make your next workout easier. Lay out your clothes, cue up a playlist, or prep a quick snack. Small prep removes big excuses.

CHAPTER 5.
THE TRICK FOR WHEN YOU SIMPLY DON'T WANT TO

When my alarm goes off in the morning, sometimes I'm already awake and excited to get going. Other times, I lie there asking myself one simple question: "How do I want my future self to feel?" I first started asking myself that question years ago, when my children were much younger and life felt like one long to-do list. Looking back now, I realize that was the season that taught me the power of preparation and grace. Let me take you back to a day from that time.

The alarm goes off at 3:30 AM. I'm training for a marathon and need to run 10 miles before my husband heads out for his own workout and then to work. Once he leaves, the morning chaos begins. I've got to get my six- and eight-year-old ready for school, make breakfast, pack lunches, and sneak in a quick stretch before the day takes off. After drop-off, I homeschool my three-year-old. That includes lessons, playtime, and outdoor time because every single one is an important piece of his routine.

Sure, I could try to squeeze my miles in during his nap, but any parent knows that's a gamble. Especially when it's marathon training miles. What if this is the one day he decides not to nap? What if he wakes up right when I find my rhythm? Nap time is also prime laundry-folding time on Mondays, or maybe it's when I try to fit in writing this very book. Before I know it, nap time's over, and it's snack time, then school pick-up time for the other two kids.

Once school's out, I'm balancing three kids, two homework sessions, and two activities, dance and flag football, before dinner even hits the table. My husband is amazing when he's home, but we're still running around like two

Uber drivers with matching exhaustion. I could technically stay home when he takes our son to football, but I'll be honest, I am that mom who gets FOMO. So off I go, toddler and middle child in tow, cheering from the sidelines.

By the time we pick up my daughter from dance, it's after seven. The boys are exhausted and need snacks and my eldest needs to read aloud to us for 15 minutes. We squeeze in our nightly prayer, talk about the best part of the day, and finally, at 8:00 p.m., I get to sit for what feels like the first time since 3:30 a.m.

That's a day. And that's why I ask myself every morning, "How do I want my future self to feel?" Because if I push that workout off, the rest of the day will own me. But if I move first and I get my workout done before the sun comes up, I know that no matter what the day throws at me, I've already done something for myself. I'll be more patient, more grounded and more capable of handling the chaos with grace instead of frustration.

Here's the thing, though: sometimes, showing up for yourself does mean staying in bed. There are days when your body truly needs rest, and ignoring that is not discipline, it's disconnection. The key is learning the difference between tired and depleted. Early in your fitness journey, it's important to build consistency, which means pushing through the "I don't feel like it" days. But as you grow, you'll also learn when your body genuinely needs to recover.

For me, I know that if I can get myself out of bed and brush my teeth, I'll be fine. That's my checkpoint. Once I start moving, I'm ready. But sometimes, even after brushing my teeth, my body says, "Nope. Go back to bed." And I make sure to listen when that happens.

This little trick of thinking ahead to how I want my future self to feel works for more than just early mornings. If I plan to work out midday, I ask, "How do

I want to feel later when the kids are home and need me?" If I'm aiming for a nighttime session, I think, "How do I want to feel when I finally lie down to sleep?" That question shifts me out of the moment and into a place of purpose.

Funny story, I came up with this method on my own one day, lying in bed, trying to talk myself into moving. A few weeks later, I heard the same idea on a podcast. I laughed out loud and I thought, "Wow, so this little mental trick really is a thing!" Turns out, it's rooted in psychology and self-regulation; the idea that if you connect to your future self, you're more likely to follow through in the present. Thinking ahead helps you zoom out from the "now" and see the ripple effect of your choices. When you imagine the peace of finishing your workout versus the frustration of skipping it, you start to realize how much control you actually have. It becomes less about forcing yourself and more about aligning with who you want to be at the end of the day.

Now, let's be real. Life doesn't care about your plans. Kids get sick, your boss needs you to stay late, the dishwasher breaks, your mood drops. Things happen. And that's okay. But if you've already decided that your workout isn't optional, you'll be ready to adapt instead of abandoning the plan completely. Sometimes that means shortening the workout, walking instead of running, or doing 10 minutes of stretching instead of 40 minutes of lifting. It still counts.

I know I talk a lot about morning workouts, and that's because they work best for me. There are fewer distractions, fewer people awake, and fewer chances for life to get in the way. But that doesn't mean it's the only way. The principle stays the same no matter when you move: visualize the version of you who already did it. When you picture yourself getting up, moving your body, and finishing strong, you're not just imagining motivation, you're creating it. Your brain starts to believe that version of you is possible, and it starts moving you toward her.

Something else that is very important to mention: The snooze button. Please, don't hit snooze more than once. Snoozing might feel like self-care, but it actually delays your momentum. If you're a chronic snoozer, try placing your alarm or phone across the room or using music that wakes you up in a good mood. I like to pick songs that lift my energy, something upbeat but not obnoxious. My husband works out early too, so we've learned that "good vibes only" applies to alarms just as much as playlists.

This mental trick of asking how you want your future self to feel is powerful because it doesn't rely on hype or discipline alone. It creates space for both motivation and grace. It lets you choose from intention instead of impulse. Some mornings, that choice will lead you straight into a great workout. Other mornings, it might lead you back under the covers for one more hour of sleep, which is okay, too. Here's the best part: once you start using this question regularly, it spills into every part of your life. I use it when I don't feel like folding laundry, cleaning the kitchen, washing my hair, or tackling a project. I ask myself, "How do I want to feel later?" And every single time, it gives me clarity. I realize that the short-term discomfort of getting started is nothing compared to the peace I'll feel once it's done. How you show up in your workouts is how you show up in your life. The same habits that get you out of bed when it's hard are the ones that help you follow through at work, with your family, and in your goals. Each small act of showing up builds confidence, not just in your body but in your ability to trust yourself.

Now that my kids are older, our mornings look a little different. Not necessarily easier, just different. The noise has shifted from snack cups and nap schedules to backpacks and sports bags, but the lesson remains the same: every season demands its own version of showing up. I still ask myself that same question each morning, "How do I want my future self to feel?" It has become a quiet mantra that grounds me no matter what life looks like. Whether I'm training for a race, recovering from loss, or simply trying to juggle another busy week, that reminder keeps me aligned. This is about awareness, grace, and choice.

Your Next Move: Build a 5-minute "bare minimum" workout you can do anywhere. Save it on a piece of paper or your phone and pull it out when motivation feels impossible.

CHAPTER 6.
FINDING THE RIGHT WORKOUT FOR YOU

Everywhere we turn, it seems there is some new workout or diet to try, all claiming to change your body in a short amount of time. Or go on social media, and there goes an aesthetically pleasing post of someone who claims to know the secret to achieving the same results. I love social media because of how I use it and who I follow. Therefore, I am not bashing it at all. But the truth is, if we do not have proper discernment, we can feel awful about ourselves after scrolling. None of us are immune to it. Then, when we feel bad, we may get discouraged. Or we try to do what we see on social media. Following something mindlessly through misinformation can be super dangerous physically and emotionally.

If you stick to the basics with exercise, especially as a beginner or someone who has not been active in a while, you can't go wrong. And I think this is the time to say: our results are widely made up of what we eat. I also know that genetics plays a role, but we must remember that we can't simply say something is because of genetics and not even try to change it. For example, high blood pressure runs in my family. Luckily, I have not experienced that. Genetics and nutrition aside, for the purposes of this chapter, you have to find the exercise that lights your soul on fire or starts as a small flame that you will nurture and grow.

If you hate running and it makes you generally averse to exercise, you probably shouldn't start your journey with running. Several people tell me they hate running but want to train for a marathon. Listen, that is a fantastic goal, and I am all for it. I know firsthand how life-changing training for a marathon can be. However, I also know that if someone hates running and has barely run, starting with training for something as physically straining and time-demanding as a marathon will probably leave them feeling burnt out and defeated. Again, I am not discouraging you from training for a goal as big as a marathon. I am saying that people tend to start hot and motivated, and then the flame quickly dies down. When that happens, they start with negative self-talk, thinking they aren't good enough. You know the saying, "Rome wasn't built in a day"? It wasn't, "…but they laid bricks down every hour." This is what we are trying to do here: create a long-lasting love story with fitness, not a hot and fiery one-night stand.

I remember thinking I should do yoga years back because it seemed like that was what everyone was doing. I thought having a yoga mat would make me pretty cool. It also looked easy; I thought 45 minutes of yoga would be a piece of cake and super unchallenging. Ha! I was quickly humbled and felt like such a fool. I couldn't do any poses and felt so defeated and weak. Every single second of every single move was so excruciating physically and mentally. I am pretty sure I did not finish the workout before telling myself, "Yoga is not my thing," and I thought that if I had to do yoga every single day forever, I would probably give up on working out altogether.

Now, here's the thing. If you're starting from an absolute point 0 and haven't done any exercising besides gym class as a child or teenager or your exercise is chasing after a toddler, many workouts might make you feel the way yoga made me feel. It did not feel good at all. Even though running is my main exercise of choice, each time I picked up running again after giving birth, the experience was pretty painful for a few weeks. It made me want to downright quit. But when we do workouts that fulfill us, there's a nice after-feeling we are left with. As each brick is laid down, we start to feel the progress and the pride that comes with it. No matter how hard the workout you choose may feel, you will know which one you should probably stick to for a while, even if it isn't pleasurable in the moment. Also, for those who may be wondering: I do not hate yoga anymore. It still is not my favorite, but I have learned to appreciate and genuinely respect what it does for my body and mind on many levels. I started liking it when I explored different types of yoga, beginning with 10 minutes instead of 30+ minutes.

So, where do you start when you're not sure which type of workout to commit to? The basics don't fail. After speaking to your doctor, of course, I recommend walking, which is something that we all may do every day. Of course, some people cannot walk, and other options can be explored. Whenever I suggest walking, some think it isn't going to be effective enough. An article by Cardiol found that walking daily helps with heart health, body composition, and even blood pressure. So much can be done with walking. You can walk on the treadmill while watching a show, or listening to music or a podcast. You can add incline to work up a sweat or utilize ankle weights, wrist weights, and/or a weighted vest. You can walk alone, enjoying the sounds of nature, or with your significant other, kids, or friends—so many possibilities.

Or maybe you prefer a stationary bike? You can go at the speed you want while still watching a show, listening to music or a podcast. For lifting and strength training, there are many combinations of different moves that may be too advanced for a beginner, but I always find myself returning to lunges, squats, and bicep curls. Proper form is also essential, so as I list these exercises, I urge you to find videos for direction or sessions with a trainer who can give you the basics and oversee your progress. I always love a good online video to ensure I am doing something correctly. I also follow various fitness programs where the trainers fully take the time to explain how an exercise should look and feel.

Another mistake people often make is trying to do what everyone else does. There are so many other exercises besides the usual ones. Maybe you're interested in tennis lessons or have friends who play basketball on the weekends. Perhaps you are intrigued by boxing. Or maybe a gym near you offers classes like Zumba or hot yoga. What about swimming? There are so many options to explore, such as African or Caribbean dancing. The key here is to have fun and look forward to the next workout. It must be mentioned that finances may be an issue, so choose what makes the most financial sense for your budget.

However, if you're part of the group that constantly says, "I don't have any money to invest in my health," I beg you to please look at where your money goes. If you're ordering food often, spending a lot on liquor, or honestly just not keeping track of your money, investing in your health is a wonderful thing to do for yourself. You don't have to give up ordering food, but I can tell you from personal experience that when I checked how much I spent ordering food for one month, I was pretty embarrassed.

We are all essentially still kids at heart. If you pay attention to children or have some of your own already, think about how they go outside and run around for a long time, not even realizing that their playing is physical exercise. When you forget that you're doing something strenuous and you get lost in the moment, you have probably found the exercise that will help you truly fall in love with fitness.

Now, please understand that if you're training for something like a marathon or bodybuilding competition, for example, this may feel a little different from workout to workout. Still, cumulatively, the feelings you're getting on your journey will help you see that you are going in the right direction. And the key here too is not to start day 1 at a high intensity that your body may not be able to keep up with, which may cause extreme fatigue or injury. This brings me to my next point: duration and days.

I hear this from many people: "I can't commit to working out every day. I try, but I don't have the time." Remember what I said about my father at the beginning of this book? He would wake up every morning and do something quickly before his shower. You do not have to work out for an hour a day every day. It's okay to start with one day a week for 10 minutes and build up from there. Again, the key here is to build slowly and have the right foundation. What would this look like? I tell everyone to start with one day a week. Commit to that for a few weeks or even months if that's what you need.

Start with 5 minutes. A 5-minute workout might sound simple and too easy, but a lot can be done in 5 minutes. Think arm circles, lunges, and jumping jacks. Five minutes is definitely enough to work up a sweat. Trust me. Now, the brain is incredible. I'm no scientist, but once you prove that you can commit to one day, your brain and body crave more. You'll find yourself going a little bit longer and adding in another day until maybe you're up to 30 minutes 3–4 days a week. You have to believe in the process and build discipline. And again, if you're engaging in an enjoyable exercise, this will be much easier.

Although we discuss working out in this chapter, what you put in your body is also essential. Therefore, I want to talk about nutrition again for a little bit. I don't want you to just fall in love with working out, but a considerable part of fitness is what you put into your body. Often, when people think "healthy eating", they immediately associate it with boring or too restrictive. Just like loving your exercise of choice, it is important to eat things you love too. What worked for me was still eating the foods I love but not overdoing it or making home-cooked versions of the meals I love. I absolutely love burgers and fries. Did I stop eating them? No. I realized making a burger at home and slicing some potatoes to put in the air fryer can be more satisfying than getting one from a restaurant. When you eat well, you function better. But if you're not into what you're eating, that's a problem. For example, I cannot stand celery. I have tried it every way you can, but it's just not my thing. So, if you do not like boring salads, don't eat boring salads!

Meal prepping can come in very handy, but if, by day 2, you're not interested in it anymore, and you're wasting food, maybe the typical way of meal prepping everything on a Sunday isn't for you. For example, some people prep for two days at a time.

There are things we have to do that we may not love. You still have to do some of those things, so I'm not saying to write off everything that you can't stand. Flirt with the idea of making something that's good for you work for you.

Your Next Move: Try one new type of movement this week. It can be a class, a walk, or a fun activity with your friends or family. Focus on how it feels, not how many calories it burns.

CHAPTER 7.
ACCOUNTABILITY

Accountability. One word, but a powerful defining factor in your journey. It helps to treat your health and fitness as a project. I know school projects aren't fun, and work projects can bring anxiety and stress. But this is your personal project that will benefit you both now and in the long run. Let's use the example of a school project.

If you're given a project to carry out, it would be a little tricky if you just jumped right in without a plan for direction and to help keep you accountable. Accountability is the backbone of your health project. What exactly is accountability by definition? The Webster dictionary defines it as "an obligation or willingness to accept responsibility for one's actions." What would that look like on a health and fitness journey? It would mean taking responsibility for everything you do, from your workouts to your nutrition and everything in between.

You can hold yourself accountable in many ways. Something that truly helps me is writing down my specific goals, whether I write them down with pen and paper, have them in a notepad on my phone, or type them up and print them out. I need to see my goal, not just in one spot. Gail Matthews (2007) found that those who write down their goals are much more likely to achieve them than those who don't. I also post my workout schedule by my closet and near my calendar. Both are places I walk by often and glance at every single day. For example, every race I have trained for since becoming a distance runner has a goal. Whether the goal is "have fun and do your best" or "finish in XYZ time," it is written down, typed up, and posted on my wall. Even my running playlist has the goal time listed on there. There needs to be a constant reminder of what you promised yourself you would do. Actually seeing what I am trying to achieve is a way to keep me accountable every day.

I didn't think this next tip would help me, but it has helped immensely. On my fitness social media page, I sometimes post about my workout goals. For example, a quick picture of my workout clothes laid out, with something along the lines of "Workout clothes ready to go! Early workout planned!" I cannot bring myself to skip a workout knowing that I told the world (or the few people who see it) that I plan on doing something. Be selective, though, with what is comfortable for you if you go this route. Leaving some things to the imagination, I do not post a goal time I want to race in.

Your goal doesn't have to be posted on social media; you can also have an accountability partner. Someone you know will hold you to what you say. Do not confuse an accountability partner with someone who magically makes you do what you say. I've sent wake-up calls to people who did not answer or had an excuse anyway. In the end, it comes down to you; everything else to help you is extra. If your accountability partner works out with you, that is even more amazing. There are so many different groups you have access to in order to find someone; it doesn't need to be someone you know personally. Or start a fun challenge with people you work with or other parents at school pickup. You can get creative and make accountability a fun process.

Treat yourself! Pause though. When I say treat yourself, it doesn't necessarily mean something that would cause you to backtrack on your progress. When I hear the word treat, my brain instantly thinks of indulging in delicious foods and goodies. I am all for celebrating the wins, but make sure you know yourself because this can be trial and error. Sometimes, I reach a goal and celebrate by ordering my favorite food. But doing that can lead me down the road of eating unhealthy for a whole weekend and sometimes even a few days into the next week. Something I find more helpful is to buy myself a new workout item of clothing. Who doesn't love new workout clothes? Again, this can be tricky if you're also working on spending habits, so be careful. Another example of a treat and a free one? Let's say I did well with my sleep goal of sleeping for over 7 hours a few times a week; I may loosen up for a night and stay up reasonably late watching some of my favorite shows or a great movie. Again, let me reiterate that I am not saying that treating yourself should feel like you have been depriving yourself. My way of eating, for example, is eating everything I love in moderation but ensuring that most of my nutrition is generally beneficial for my goals.

When it comes to accountability, it is also beneficial to have a backup plan. However, while it is wonderful to have something to fall back on in case the first route didn't work or isn't working, you need to be cautious not to automatically default to that backup plan. Sometimes, a backup plan can become a crutch. For example, you aim to wake up at 5:00 AM to work out before work all week, but you keep snoozing your alarm every time it goes off because you have a backup plan to work out later in the day. It shouldn't become an easy way out.

Another example is that you meal-prepped for the whole week, but by the second day, you're not eating any of it, and the food is going to waste. Now, did you actually cook things you like? Are you eating out at work and ignoring the fact that you have food already? As mentioned in the previous chapter, maybe meal prepping for the whole week isn't for you, and you should cook for a few days at a time. Or perhaps you must reevaluate other habits preventing you from reaching your fullest potential with meal prepping.

Let's go back to the project analogy. When you have the foundation of how you're going to do what you said you would do, how you're going to do it, and precisely what you're going to do, you're setting the stage for the best possible outcome. Sometimes, you won't want to wake up and work out. Okay, maybe you'll feel that way most of the time. Often, the motivation we are looking for isn't there until we get started. It's vital to remember that when you don't want to do something.

Did you always want to write those papers and complete those projects in high school? I am going to take a guess and assume no. But when you took the time to prepare (if you did), you probably realized how much easier it was to have the foundation ready and a plan for how you would do what you said you would do; it makes it all feel a little less daunting. We do not want this health and fitness journey to feel daunting, so minimizing uncertainty as much as possible is vital. It feels good to have all of the preliminary guesswork figured out. Alarm, set. Clothes laid out. Supplements are on the kitchen counter, and your workout is already clearly written down.

Part of accountability is also revising your original plan to ensure that it still aligns with what you are trying to achieve. Different seasons of life can bring on different criteria needed for your goals. This is similar to a backup plan, but it's really just making sure that everything you are doing stays how it is or is tweaked if necessary. It doesn't necessarily mean doing less either. For example, depending on the season of life I am in, I may be able to add longer workouts to my schedule or extra stretching or even not worry about meal prepping because I have the time to cook all my meals fresh that day. We are constantly changing, whether we see it or not. I love to wake up early to work out but sometimes I can get more done right after dropping the kids off at school without rushing as much as I would with an earlier workout.

Being a novice or making a comeback in taking control of your health and fitness already presents enough challenges, so try to minimize as many as you can. The way you hold yourself accountable will continually be of great importance. While it may be easy the first week to do what you said you would do, there will be harder and more challenging days and days when you just want to quit. Do not quit; hold yourself accountable.

Your Next Move: Tell one person your workout goal for the week. Ask them to check in, or even better, invite them to join you for extra encouragement.

CHAPTER 8.
GOAL SETTING & MEASURING

Throw out the scales! I'm kidding, but they can make you feel like you've failed before you've even started. Scales can be a beneficial tool as long as you understand there is WAY more to defining your success than your weight.

Let me be fully transparent: I do use my scales at certain points, especially when I'm working toward weight loss, such as after having children. However, I keep in mind that many factors can influence the number it presents. If I haven't used the bathroom yet for the day (ahem, had a number 2), the number will be higher. If I'm wearing clothes, it will be higher. If I haven't breastfed yet, you better believe it, it's higher. And as a woman, don't forget that where you are in your cycle plays a significant role. So again, the number on the scales can be handy, but I suggest you combine it with other ways to measure your success.

Let me share with you some other ways to measure your success. Firstly, measurements. Someone can weigh 180 pounds today as they begin their journey, and then a few weeks later weigh the same but have different measurements. If you have never measured yourself before, I suggest watching a tutorial video and/or having someone help you properly. There are many different measurements you can take. Here are the most common ones: bust, waist, hips. However, you can take it even further: arms (bicep area), thighs, neck. Write these numbers down (in inches or centimeters, whatever you prefer) and keep them safe. As I would suggest with the scale, do not take measurements every day.

I like to do this once a week at most, but it's even better if you wait a little longer—think every 2–4 weeks. You will find which works better for you. Some people can take measurements, notice no change, and keep going. Others may take measurements and not see a change, start negative self-talk, and take some steps back. There is another side to this: seeing the numbers you want and then getting very comfortable OR seeing the numbers you wish to and getting so excited you go harder. I have experienced all of these situations at some point. You might have as well, or maybe you will. The critical thing to remember is that change will happen when you keep going and stick to the plan. The results will come if you eat nutritious meals and put in the gym work.

That said, progress doesn't always look the same for everyone. There are seasons where effort doesn't translate immediately into visible change, and that doesn't mean you're doing something wrong. Factors like stress, recovery, and hormonal shifts, can influence how the body responds. This is why it's important to measure success in more than one way.

Another beneficial way to measure your progress requires no math. Yay! It's all about how you're feeling. How do your clothes feel on your body? How do you feel mentally? How do you feel at the end of the day when you would typically be fatigued, and how do you feel after carrying in the groceries?

One thing I would advise against is buying clothes in a smaller size on purpose and aiming to fit into them. The issue with this is that all your focus will be on that item of clothing rather than the overall picture. I have witnessed so many people work toward fitting into that dress that they bought three sizes too small and then developed the most negative outlook on health and fitness because they didn't fit into it three months later. This is a surefire way NOT to fall in love with fitness.

I also want to mention holding onto clothes we used to fit. Listen, I may work out, eat well most of the time, and be back down to pre-pregnancy weight, but my body has changed. It took me years to let go of some of my pre-pregnancy clothes. When you carry a child or get older in general, your body changes. It doesn't matter that you lost 30 pounds, some clothes won't fit the same anymore. I remember feeling so frustrated when I was back down to pre-pregnancy weight after my first baby, but those low-rise jeans I loved so much still couldn't zip. Birthing a baby can change your body in many different ways. A few years ago, I decided to try on everything I had pre-baby and finally let go of the ones that wouldn't fit me anymore. Is this what happens to everyone? Not at all, but I want to put this reality out there so that you can relay the message if it does happen to you or someone you know.

I recommend wearing the clothes you usually wear and noticing how they start to fit differently after starting your fitness journey. You might notice that your jeans were much easier to zip, that you feel more comfortable sitting down, or that maybe you need a belt when you didn't before. These are all things we call "non-scale victories." Another terrific non-scale victory is being able to carry many grocery bags in at once without struggling. This is one of my favorites because I love carrying heavy things without feeling exhausted afterward. Another one of my favorites is giving one of my kids a piggyback ride while holding another. It instantly makes me thank my workout regimen and has nothing to do with my appearance.

Another way to measure progress is with photos. Taking pictures is very hard for some people, as they're usually wearing minimal clothing, something tight, or a bathing suit. It doesn't matter that these pictures are simply for them. Something about stripping down and taking real footage can leave some feeling guilty or embarrassed about their appearance. But let me tell you, this is a powerful tool. When you see your day 1 picture compared to day 100, for example, it is mind-blowing. Also, knowing that you're going to get vulnerable again and take new pictures in a few weeks can really keep the momentum going. After having my third baby, I ran a challenge group where we documented our progress by taking photos of ourselves. Even though I saw myself in the mirror daily, I never saw how I looked in photos. Sure, the camera may add a few pounds, but between the pictures and my measurements, I knew I had work to do. My body had just given birth to my third child; it was normal. But I was still shocked when comparing my before and later pictures. I don't like to say before/after pictures because, again, this is a never-ending journey. Regardless, seeing my results and all my clients' results in the group was lovely. So, when you take your pictures, use them as fuel to remember where you are headed.

I have mentioned a few points that seem to deal with how we look externally. Working out is so much more than appearance, though. So. Much. More. Many people start working out because they want to change their appearance. Many people continue working out because they realize it keeps them feeling mentally stable and balanced. This became much more apparent to me after becoming a mother. The mental and emotional benefits of working out showed themselves before (during college, graduate school, stress with wedding planning, random down days, marriage). Becoming a mother, though, was when they became impossible to ignore. I started noticing that my children feed off my energy as a mom. If I am having a bad day, they don't seem like themselves, even if I am still patient and attentive. We are all entitled to have our down days. Not everyone has children or dreams of having them, but down days are a little different when you have small humans to care for. And it's not just with kids: our energy, mood, and emotional regulation affect all relationships at home, at work, and elsewhere.

Often when people watch me interact with my children, they comment on my high level of patience. First and foremost, my mother is the most patient woman I have ever met in my life, so I do take some of that from her. However,

I started to notice that when my health and fitness is not a priority, I don't feel like myself, I am not fun and I am not that pleasant. From the outside, maybe a bystander wouldn't notice. I know myself, though, and when I am operating at my best. I tell everyone that I am the mother and wife that I am because of how I take care of my body (and my mind).

Another way to measure your success is by tracking your metrics. Maybe this week you do bicep curls with 5lb weights but a month from now you're using 10lb weights. That is huge! Or if you're training for a race, maybe you ran a mile in 14 minutes the first time you tried but, in a few months, you got that time down to a 12-minute mile. These numbers tell you so much more than your weight alone could.

Let's talk about sleep quality. Have you ever noticed how your sleep is different when you're exercising and eating well? When you treat your body right and get in some fitness, your sleep quality changes too, even during those dreaded winter months. I just sleep so much better at night when I am taking care of my body. Sleep issues aside, such as sleep apnea, you will notice that the quality of your sleep improves when you're looking after yourself. I see a huge difference after drinking alcohol, for example. My heart rate is higher during my tracked sleep, and my sleep is not peaceful. I also wake up in the night and take ages to fall back asleep.

Speaking of heart rate, that is something else that can greatly improve after taking consistent care of your health. I took a health psychology class in undergraduate school, and became a little obsessed with my heart rate and VO2 max! You can track your resting heart rate, which reflects how healthy your heart is, and your VO2 max, which reflects how efficiently your body uses oxygen. During consistent training, my resting heart rate often drops into the 40s and 50s, which is a sign that my endurance is improving. It fluctuates if I've had a weekend of fun, but it usually balances back out. And along with that, my VO2 max increases when I am more fit. Just remember, everyone's numbers are different, so use these as guides, not grades.

Taking all these ways to track your progress into account will show you the effects of your hard work. If you want to enjoy the process, know that things can take longer than you may have imagined. Having different ways to measure will help you mentally and give you momentum. It is so easy to just keep focusing on the end goal instead of taking everything into account. The end goal is wonderful but keeping sight of everything you are doing to lead you there is honestly more wonderful. Sometimes, the end goal takes longer or sometimes it changes. What should not change is the pride you feel for yourself as you overcome everything along the way.

Your Next Move: Write down one short-term fitness goal you can reach in the next two weeks. Put it somewhere visible, like your fridge or planner, so it stays in front of you.

CHAPTER 9.
CONTROL WHAT YOU CAN

Things will happen that are out of your control, weekly if not daily. Something I see often is that people tend to have an all-or-nothing attitude. If they can't get all their workouts and healthy meals in, they quit and throw away the entire day, week, month, and even year. We can't control every single factor around us, as much as we want to.

Picture this: you've arrived at work, and a coworker bought delicious donuts for the office. You told yourself you weren't going to eat one, but now you've had three. Another coworker suggests ordering lunch even though you packed your own. At this point, you can either get back on track with your healthy lunch or throw the day away and order out. The better decision is clear, but it's also hard when that inner voice starts whispering, "You already messed up. Might as well start over tomorrow."

That's the danger of the all-or-nothing mindset. Once you tell yourself you've failed, it becomes easier to spiral. What could have been a single decision becomes a pattern. The real power is in catching yourself mid-spiral and pausing, breathing, and choosing again. You don't need perfection to make progress. You just need the awareness to turn things around in the middle of the mess.

You can even prepare for things like this ahead of time. If you know your co-workers like to order lunch once a week, plan for it. Enjoy it without guilt, and then return to your rhythm the next day. The goal isn't control over everything; it's control over how you respond when things go off script.

Let's look at another example. You've started a new fitness program and did amazing for week one. Then week two hits, and you oversleep on Monday. You have 15 minutes before work but skip the workout entirely, telling yourself you'll double up tomorrow (which I don't typically recommend). Then Tuesday comes and you miss it again. That "I'll just start Monday" mentality creeps in, and suddenly it's been two weeks. Missing one workout isn't failure, but giving it power over your momentum is. If you oversleep, use the 15 minutes you do have. Do half the workout. Stretch. Go for a walk after work. The goal is to stay connected to your routine, so it never disappears. This is what controlling what you can looks like.

Running and motherhood taught me a fundamental lesson: your day will rarely go as planned. Kids wake up early, deadlines shift, weather ruins your outdoor plans, dinner is ruined, someone gets sick. But essentially, your mindset determines whether those things stop you or simply redirect you. The people who stay consistent aren't the ones who never miss a day; they're the ones who refuse to stay down when things go wrong.

When my kids were younger, there were so many days when the timing just didn't work. My perfectly planned morning would collapse, and I'd have a choice: give up, or pivot. I learned to go for a run with the jogging stroller or get in a 20-minute solo walk on the treadmill, or a short workout before bed. Those small wins added up. They reminded me that control doesn't always look like the plan you made. It's how you adapt when the plan falls apart.

The "control what you can" mindset is also deeply emotional. You can't always control your stress levels, grief, or the curveballs life throws, but you can control your response to them. You can choose how you speak to yourself when things go off course. Although difficult, you can choose to stop the negative spiral. It is vital to be able to master your reaction to what's outside your hands.

I also want to explore a fascinating and sometimes concerning topic: the "New Year, New Me" mindset. I've been there multiple times. I'm not knocking anyone who wants to start something new on January 1st. Starting is always worth celebrating and I will stand by that. But if you wait for the perfect moment to begin, you train yourself to believe that success only happens under perfect conditions. And perfect conditions don't exist.

Dr. Shah writes that about 77% of people who make New Year's goals fail within the first few weeks. That is a huge and alarming number. It's exciting to set goals, but without a plan, the motivation fades. If you've ever been part of a gym, you've seen it. The gyms are packed in January with no room to breathe, but then they become half-empty by February. The brain loves novelty, but it struggles with consistency. So, start before the new year. Start before Monday. Start in the middle of chaos. That's when your habits stick.

Many people say they don't want to begin a health or fitness regimen during the holidays because of all the food and parties. Honestly? That's one of the best times to start. It teaches discipline without deprivation. It shows you that your habits can live alongside real life. When you start during the hard seasons, you prove to yourself that you can keep going when things aren't ideal—and that's the kind of resilience that lasts.

Here's what that looks like in my world: Before the holidays, when the kids start school in September, life feels like a tornado. There's homework, sports, parent meetings, dinners, laundry, and the endless list that comes with parenting. But I can control getting my workout done. That's my constant. During the holidays, I still eat the Halloween candy, enjoy Thanksgiving leftovers for a few days, and make cookies with my kids, which includes me eating the cookie dough right along with them. But I don't abandon my workouts, my water intake or my morning routines. Even if it's a lighter workout, I stay connected to movement.

That's how you build a rhythm that lasts. It may bend, but it doesn't break. When January rolls around, you won't feel like you are starting over. You will feel like you are simply continuing. Sure, you might be tired, or your body may feel heavy during workouts from all the festivities, but you will still start the year with momentum, not guilt.

Even though this book is focused on health and fitness, this idea applies to every area of life. The thing about starting now rather than waiting for the perfect day, week, or year is that you're training your brain to follow through no matter what. Life won't slow down to make room for your goals. You have to move forward in the middle of it.

Control what you can. Let the rest go. If you can drink your water, do your workout, speak kindly to yourself, and get some sleep, you've already succeeded. When you start to notice that progress isn't about how perfectly you perform but how consistently you come back, you'll realize something powerful: control isn't the enemy of freedom; it's the foundation of peace.

Your Next Move: Pick one thing you can fully control this week, whether that's water intake, daily steps, or bedtime.

CHAPTER 10.
MENTAL HEALTH AND FITNESS

It would be a huge disservice not to include a section on mental health in this book. Yes, eating well and exercising have countless benefits for your mind, but that's not where we're starting. Before we talk about how movement improves mental health, we have to discuss what stops so many people from ever moving in the first place: the mental block.

That mental block is heavy. It's the invisible weight that keeps you from lacing up your shoes, cooking the meal you planned, or believing you're capable of lasting change. It shows up differently for everyone. For some, it's fear. The fear of failing, fear of starting over, or fear of not being good enough. For others, it's depression, anxiety, or the constant loop of negative self-talk that whispers, "Why bother?" Sometimes, it's being stuck in the past, holding on to who you used to be or how your body used to look. Other times, it's the mental exhaustion that comes from simply being a human with too much to carry.

All of these things are real, and if any of them sound familiar, please know that you're not broken. You're human. But that doesn't mean you have to stay stuck. Let's take a closer look at what these blocks can look like and how to start moving through them.

FEAR OF FAILING

Fear is often the biggest obstacle to success, as I've mentioned several times throughout this book. It can stop you before you even take the first step. Starting again can feel terrifying, especially if you've tried before and quit, or if you're afraid of what others will think if you don't follow through.

The truth is, a healthy lifestyle doesn't give you instant results. It's not like studying for a test or trying a new recipe and seeing success pretty instantly. Fitness is a long-term relationship with yourself. That delay between effort and reward can feel extremely discouraging, and that's when fear creeps in.

What breaks fear is action. Not motivation, not waiting for the perfect day. Action. One small choice in your favor today is proof that you're capable. Maybe that means putting on your shoes, prepping your lunch, or pressing play on a 10-minute workout. You can't control the timeline, but you can control your consistency. And when fear tells you you're not enough, remind yourself that showing up is proof that you already are.

DEPRESSION AND THE WEIGHT OF IT ALL

The World Health Organization reports that depression is about 50% more common in women than in men, and around 1 in 10 pregnant or postpartum women experience it. When you're in that space, even getting out of bed can feel like climbing a mountain. So, the thought of adding workouts and meal prep on top of everything? It can feel impossible.

This isn't about minimizing that reality, it's about acknowledging that movement can help you cope when you're ready. Research shows that even small amounts of movement can lift mood and lessen symptoms. But getting there takes time.

If you're navigating depression, take things one micro-step at a time. Maybe one day you just think about working out. The next, you put on your clothes but never press play. It's progress even if it seems minor. The next day, maybe you move for 5 minutes. That's still something. Healing and fitness are both non-linear journeys. Some days, you'll feel strong. Other days, the most courageous thing you'll do is get dressed. Give yourself credit for that.

And please, if you're struggling, talk to someone. A therapist, a doctor, a trusted friend or all three. Fitness is powerful, but it's not meant to replace professional help. It is meant to work alongside it.

THE BATTLE WITH NEGATIVE SELF-TALK

Negative self-talk is one of the biggest roadblocks to growth. It's that inner critic that tells you you'll always look this way, or that you'll never be able to stick with anything. And when you've spent years speaking to yourself that way, it becomes a hard habit to break.

One of the most effective tools for this is Cognitive Behavioral Therapy (CBT), a practice that helps you interrupt negative thoughts before they shape your behavior. Instead of letting your thoughts spiral, you challenge them.

For example:

Negative thought: "There's no point in working out. I'll never see results."

Reframe: "Even if I don't see results right away, I'm doing something good for myself. Change takes time."

Constantly work on speaking to yourself like someone you love. Sometimes, that even means calling out your own mental tricks. "I'll start tomorrow." "I've already messed up the week." These are stories your brain tells you to stay comfortable. But the moment you notice them, you're gaining power over your self-talk. You can't always silence the negative voice, but you can decide not to let it lead.

HEALING THE RELATIONSHIP WITH YOUR BODY

So much of how we approach health begins in childhood with what we saw, what we were told, and how we were treated. Maybe you were bullied for your body. Maybe you grew up watching adults constantly criticize theirs. Or maybe you were only praised when you looked a certain way. Those experiences shape the way you care for yourself now, and sometimes, without realizing it, they keep you from trying again.

It's time to unlearn that conditioning. You're not defined by who you were or what was said about you, and the beauty here is that you get to write a new story about what strength, beauty, and confidence look like.

I had to learn this. After pregnancy, I developed diastasis recti, a separation of the abdominal muscles that left me feeling like my body had betrayed me. It made me look several months pregnant by the end of the day and I still deal with it from time to time. But working on healing it taught me one of the most important lessons of all: recovery isn't just physical, it's also mental. It's learning to forgive your body for changing and to thank it for carrying you through. You may not be able to "bounce back," but you can rebuild stronger inside and out. The unforeseen challenge of diastasis recti really taught me so many lessons about body acceptance, along with hard work.

MENTAL WEAKNESS VS. MENTAL STRENGTH

Being mentally strong does not mean you won't struggle. But you will learn how to show up through the mental struggles. Mental weakness can look like needing validation to start, quitting when it gets uncomfortable, or using small setbacks as reasons to stop. Strength, on the other hand, is built in those exact moments when you choose to act anyway.

When I ran my first marathon, I thought I had prepared for everything physically, mentally, and emotionally. But around mile 15, I hit a wall. My body was fine, but my mind was loud. "You've done enough. Stop now." That day taught me that the brain is both your biggest limiter and your greatest weapon. I overcame it physically by crossing the finish line, but I did not overcome the marathon mentally. I walked a lot and I let doubt take over.

Before my second marathon, I trained my mind as intentionally as my body. I practiced mantras, visualized difficult moments, and reminded myself daily why I started. When mile 15 came again, I didn't walk. I ran stronger all the way to the finish line. That's the power of building mental strength: having the ability to keep moving despite the fear.

EVOLVING BEYOND OLD VERSIONS OF YOURSELF

One of the hardest parts of change is letting go of who you used to be. You might find yourself thinking, "I used to be so fit," or "I'll never be that person again." But growth means becoming someone new, not returning to someone old. You're allowed to evolve. Your body changes, and your circumstances change along with your goals. And that's not failure, that's life. What matters is that you're still choosing to show up for yourself.

Whether you're getting back into fitness after years away, recovering from pregnancy, or simply redefining what wellness means to you now, remember this: the goal isn't to "get back" to anything. It's to move forward with grace, strength, and gratitude for where you are now.

You can't separate mental health from physical health. They move together. Strength isn't just about lifting weights or running faster. It's about lifting your thoughts and believing that you deserve to feel well, to move freely, and to rebuild even when life feels heavy.

Your Next Move: Use movement as medicine. Plan one workout this week where your only goal is to feel lighter mentally, not to hit a number or personal best.

CHAPTER 11.
SELF-FULFILLING PROPHECY

Whether you believe you can or cannot do something will often become what happens. That's the heart of a self-fulfilling prophecy. What you think about a situation ends up shaping how it turns out because your thoughts influence your behavior. As psychology writer Kendra Cherry explains, "A self-fulfilling prophecy is an expectation or belief that can influence your behaviors, thus causing the belief to come true." In other words, your actions start aligning with whatever story your brain has already decided to believe. I have always been intrigued by the idea of self-fulfilling prophecies.

This can work for you or against you, depending on how your mind is wired. An August 2016 study published in the Journal of Behavioral Medicine found that participants who already held a positive mindset toward exercise experienced greater benefits after a single workout. Their thoughts literally enhanced the results.

So, let's put this into a real-life context.

Imagine someone just invested in a brand-new home gym. Before it's even set up, they're saying things like, "I'll never use this," or "This is such a waste of money; I should've just stuck with a gym membership." Does this sound familiar to you? Here's the twist. They've never actually used that gym membership either. Because they expect failure, their actions start to match. They might skip reading the instruction manual for their new gym equipment, forget to lay out workout clothes, or constantly "run out of time." Maybe they even sign up for another gym just to justify why the home setup collects dust.

I've met so many people like this; people with beautiful home gyms filled with expensive equipment that never gets touched. We actually got our Peloton bike very cheaply, I might add, from someone who bought it new but never even used it. People say, "Having equipment here makes it harder for me to work out because it's right there." Huh? I think there is mental pressure that can come with having equipment constantly visible. For some people, seeing it every day becomes a reminder of what they haven't done yet, which can create guilt, avoidance, or an all-or-nothing mindset. Instead of feeling motivating, it can feel heavy or overwhelming, so they disengage altogether.

For other people, the barrier isn't the equipment or setup itself, but the story they tell themselves around it. Some people say they genuinely need a gym environment to stay consistent, but still have a gym membership they don't use. I think the setup becomes an easy place to place blame rather than addressing the real issue: consistency.

I get it. For a long time, I was in that same mindset. I didn't understand the appeal of working out at home until I had kids. We're all in different seasons with different comfort levels. But at some point, you have to call your own bluff. If every solution comes with a new excuse, the problem might not be the setup. It might be the story you're telling yourself.

Let's be honest, there will always be a convenient excuse. "It's too cold." "I'm too tired." "I'll start Monday." Even after all these years, I have days pretty often when I don't feel like getting up, when the bed feels too good and the motivation just isn't there. That's normal. The key is remembering that even if you don't feel it right now, doing something—anything—is better than letting another day slip by.

Here's another common example. Someone who's struggled with their nutrition for years finally decides to make a change. They fill up the fridge with healthy foods and feel hopeful… until day one hits. They wake up and think, "What's the point? I've failed before, and I'll fail again." Those thoughts set the tone for everything that follows. They skip breakfast, grab takeout for lunch, order pizza for dinner, and by the end of the night, they've convinced themselves they were right all along. "See? I knew I couldn't do it."

These examples might sound like a stretch, but they happen in small ways too. The self-fulfilling prophecy doesn't just show up in big life changes; it sneaks in during everyday moments. It's the voice that says, "I can't lift that weight," or "I'll never stick with this routine." And when you listen to it, you prove yourself right. The good news? You can flip it.

Just like negative thoughts create negative outcomes, positive ones can shape success. Think of it as rewriting the narrative in your own head. Similar to cognitive behavioral therapy, it's about catching the unhelpful thought and replacing it with something better. Not delusion but belief. I always say a small dose of delusion mixed with determination is the secret ingredient to extraordinary outcomes. Okay, I didn't always say that, but I have taught myself to think that way.

So, let's revisit that home gym example. The reversed version goes like this: you're setting up your equipment and instead of doubting yourself, you tell yourself, "This time will be different. Even if I miss a day, it doesn't mean I've failed. I'm human." The night before your workout, you set out your clothes and decide exactly what you'll do. When the alarm goes off, sure, you hesitate for a second, but then you picture how you'll feel after you move. You remind yourself why you started. You show up, you sweat, and afterward you look in the mirror, smile and say, "I am so proud of myself."

That's how it starts. One workout, one choice, one positive thought at a time. Not perfect, but consistent. Each time you prove yourself right in a good way, your confidence grows. Before you know it, you've built evidence that you can do hard things. You've changed your self-image from "I can't" to "I always find a way."

The same goes for the person working on nutrition. Maybe she says, "I haven't been showing up the way I want to, but that ends now." She shops for groceries, plans out meals, and gives herself permission to enjoy treats in moderation. When she slips up, she doesn't spiral. She adjusts. She celebrates progress, not perfection. Each week she feels a little stronger, her clothes fit differently, and she has more energy. That momentum builds, and suddenly, she's no longer trying to become "the type of person who eats healthy." She *is* that person.

This is how the self-fulfilling prophecy becomes a tool for self-care instead of self-sabotage. You start to see that the people who seem so disciplined or "fit" aren't perfect. They have the same thoughts and temptations as everyone else. The difference is that they don't let those thoughts drive their behavior. They interrupt them, reframe them, and keep going.

I've had my own moments of self-fulfilling prophecies outside of fitness, too. There have been times when I thought, "I'll probably mess this up," and then, somehow, I did because I was already halfway convinced I would. But then I began applying what I'd learned through fitness, changing the internal dialogue first, and everything else followed. It takes practice and repetition.

When you start feeding yourself new thoughts, your actions start catching up. Maybe at first you don't fully believe the new narrative, and that's okay. You keep repeating it anyway. "I'm consistent." "I'm strong." "I'm capable." You keep proving it to yourself until the belief becomes truth.

The real secret is consistency and reminding yourself daily that you have the power to decide what your story will be. Because the mind is incredibly obedient and it will follow the direction you give it. If you say, "I'll never be fit," your brain says, "Okay, let's make that true." But if you say, "I'm becoming stronger every day," your brain starts finding ways to support that. That's why awareness is everything. The next time you catch yourself saying, "I can't," pause and ask if that thought is helping you. If it's not, change it. Rewrite it. It might feel uncomfortable at first, but eventually, the new story becomes second nature.

You don't have to have every part of your journey figured out. You just need to pay attention to what you're telling yourself and choose to speak life into your goals. A self-fulfilling prophecy can destroy your progress, or it can build it. The choice is ultimately yours.

Your Next Move: Write one statement you want to believe about yourself in fitness ("I am consistent," "I am strong"). Stick it on a mirror and/or repeat it out loud before your next workout.

CHAPTER 12.
GRIEF IN MOTION

Fitness isn't just for the good days. It's for the days you don't think you can get out of bed. It's not only about chasing goals; sometimes it's about surviving loss. Movement can be a rope when life feels like it's pulling you under.

When I started writing this book, my mom, Manette, was still here. She passed away suddenly in the middle of my writing process, and it changed everything. My mom wasn't just a part of my life, she was a part of my fitness journey. She watched my kids so I could run, she asked about my workouts, she made sure I had space to breathe. Losing her was like losing a piece of my foundation.

In these first weeks without her, movement has felt very different. Some days, it feels impossible. Other days, it's the only thing keeping me upright. I was on a run when I found out she was gone. One moment my steps felt light and familiar, and the next, my heart was pounding for an entirely different reason. That moment fused running with the worst news of my life. My body remembered the shock, the drop in my stomach, the rush of adrenaline, and the way my heart seemed to race out of rhythm.

The next day, I could barely make it a mile. I cried from the first step to the last, but that mile was everything. It was proof that I could still move when it felt like my world had stopped. A few days later, I managed three miles and even felt a spark of strength return, but it didn't last. For a while, some runs were just a single slow mile that I struggled through. Other runs felt lighter and carried me farther. This has reminded me that grief is not linear. Some days your body feels capable, and others it feels like you're dragging every step through quicksand.

This chapter is not just about my experience. It's here to help you keep moving in ways that feel good, healthy, and possible when life has knocked you flat. Whether you're grieving a person, a relationship, or a dream, these tools can help you move forward without forcing yourself to "get over it."

Here are some tips I have compiled, which I hope will help you, too.

LOWER THE BAR ON WHAT "COUNTS"

In grief, even small tasks can feel monumental. On some days, a short walk, light stretching, or a few minutes of deep breathing may be all you can manage, and there is nothing wrong with that. Movement isn't about intensity right now; it's about keeping the connection between you and your body.

You might:

- Walk for 5–10 minutes outside.

- Try gentle mobility or yoga in your living room.

- Do a breathing exercise before bed.

- Expect Emotional Release Mid-Workout

Grief lives in the body, not just the mind. You might cry during a run, feel anger during a lift, or need to stop suddenly because emotions hit hard. Let it happen. You're not "doing it wrong." In fact, you're doing it exactly right.

Tip: Keep tissues or a towel nearby, and don't feel the need to explain tears to anyone.

LISTEN FOR THE REST AND PUSH SIGNALS

There will be days your body whispers, "Move." Other days it will plead, "Please rest." Both are valid. Rest days are for mercy and healing, not laziness. Push days are for release, reminding yourself that you can carry heavy things.

ANCHOR YOURSELF WITH ROUTINE

Grief is unpredictable, but a rough structure can give you something steady to hold onto. If you normally work out in the mornings, try to keep that time, even if you only do 10 minutes. The predictability can feel like safety when everything else feels uncertain.

MOVE WITH OTHERS, ESPECIALLY YOUR KIDS

Grief can make you want to isolate yourself, but sometimes moving with others helps you reconnect to life. For me, that often meant working out with my kids. We've done living room circuits, runs at the park or track, and yoga together. It wasn't just about staying active, it was about letting them see that moving your body is a healthy way to process hard emotions.

Why it helps:

- You get companionship without pressure to talk about your feelings.

- It turns movement into a shared positive experience during a painful season.

- It shows your children (or loved ones) how to care for themselves in hard times.

PAIR MOVEMENT WITH GENTLE NOURISHMENT

Loss can disrupt eating habits. Some people may lose their appetite, others overeat and some people have a combination of both. Aim for simple, nourishing foods before and after movement so your body has the fuel to process both the workout and the emotions.

GIVE YOURSELF A LONG RUNWAY

You don't have to bounce back. Grief isn't a sprint; it's a lifelong adjustment. A true marathon. Your fitness may ebb and flow. Let that be okay. Over time, you'll find your strength looks different. In seasons of grief, strength doesn't look like pushing harder or doing more; it often looks like showing up gently, adjusting expectations, choosing movement that supports your mental health, or simply continuing.

Mental strength can be the choice to keep moving when you don't want to. Physical strength can look like shorter runs, lighter workouts, or gentler movement than before. The effort is still there because your body is moving even though it's difficult; strength is just expressed differently.

I ran my first race in September, three months after my mom passed. My body felt so heavy and I really had to keep putting one foot in front of the other and keep telling myself to finish the race. It was a very hilly and challenging 10k, but I did it.

Final Thought

Movement won't erase your grief, but it can hold you steady when nothing else does. On my hardest days, a short run, a walk outside, or a few minutes of stretching didn't make the pain disappear, but they gave me enough air to take the next step.

Grief changes you. But it can also deepen your relationship with movement, turning it from a hobby into a lifeline. Even without the phone call or text message after my run from my mother, I know that she is still with me in every mile, every breath, every finish line.

Your Next Move: Choose the gentlest form of movement you can manage this week. Even if it's stretching in bed or walking to the mailbox, let it be enough.

CHAPTER 13.
IN IT FOR THE LONG HAUL

The goal here is to do this forever in some shape or form. That's why people call it a lifestyle. It's why they say fitness is a marathon, not a sprint. Think of it like cleaning your home. If you deep clean once, it looks amazing for a few days, maybe even a few weeks, depending on the ages of your kids, but eventually dust returns, laundry piles up again, and you have to start over. Most people wouldn't say that they love cleaning, but they do it anyway because it has to be done. So, they find a way to make it enjoyable. Maybe they play music, make it a game, or focus on how satisfying it feels once it's done.

Fitness works the same way. You can eat a healthy meal one day or crush a workout and feel great afterward, but to experience real results, you have to keep going. You have to keep showing up, even on the days it doesn't feel fun or exciting. That's what turns effort into lifestyle.

I won't lie and say I'm always motivated to work out. There are mornings when I sit in bed and talk myself out of pressing "start." But after years of doing this, I know the feeling that comes after is always worth it. Still, there are rough seasons. There are stretches when everything feels heavier and progress seems slower. Especially when you're starting out, those moments can last a while. You'll question your "why." You'll wonder if it's worth it. But if you can remember the bigger picture...the reason you began in the first place, it helps. This journey isn't just about abs or endurance. It's about discipline, peace, strength, and energy. It's about the kind of life you want to live. And even the kind of life you want to exemplify for those who look up to you.

Sleep is a major part of that equation. If you're not sleeping enough, that's mistake number one. I didn't fully understand the power of sleep until I became a mother. When you're younger, you can get away with short nights and still bounce back. I remember going out with friends, getting home late, and showing up for work on three hours of rest. Those days are long gone. Now, as a mom of three, I can't play myself like that. It catches up to me too quickly. If you're in a season of life where sleep just isn't consistent—new parenthood, a demanding job, unpredictable nights—give yourself grace. Take the rest when you can. For everyone else who has the opportunity to sleep but stays up scrolling, binging shows, or "just one more episode"-ing their way past midnight, you're only making things harder. Sleep isn't optional. It's a vital part of performance, focus, and recovery. You can't pour from an empty cup, and you definitely can't lift, run, or grow from one either.

When I start to feel unmotivated or stuck, one of the most powerful resets for me is fueling my mind. There are times when I've been working out consistently, eating well, and getting rest, but something still feels off. I used to push through it without questioning why, but now I recognize that it usually means my mindset needs attention. Years ago, I would have reached for a physical book for inspiration, but between kids, work, and life, my reading time disappeared. It took me forever to finish a single book. Then one day, a friend recommended a podcast episode for my commute. I hesitated, but I listened and I was instantly hooked. The episode was short, just 20 minutes, but it gave me so much perspective. That's how I discovered that podcasts and audiobooks could be fuel too.

Since then, I've listened to everything from short motivational messages to long interviews about parenting, marriage, faith, and mindset. It doesn't always have to be about fitness to impact my fitness. Sometimes, hearing someone talk about courage or perseverance lights the same fire that helps me lace up my shoes the next day. Now, if I go too long without listening to something positive, I can feel it. My mood dips, my focus scatters, and my drive starts to fade. You don't need to listen for hours every day. Even 10 minutes of encouragement while driving or folding laundry can shift your energy and remind you why you started.

If you haven't already, find voices that speak to you. The right book or podcast can act like a coach in your ear or a quiet reminder that you're not doing this alone. It's an easy way to stay inspired and build mental strength without needing extra time in your day.

Another piece that has shaped my journey in ways I never expected is faith. Not everyone reading this will be religious, and that's okay. But if you have any kind of spiritual belief, I encourage you to bring that into your fitness journey. For me, faith and fitness have become deeply connected. When I'm running, I feel closest to God. It's the quiet moments between steps when I can feel peace wash over me. There have been times I wanted to stop mid-run, when quitting felt like the only option, but I prayed instead. I've had countless runs where I've asked for strength, and somehow, it came full force. It's hard to explain, but I've seen enough signs to know those moments weren't coincidence.

Over time, my workouts became more than physical. They became conversations with myself, with God, with the strength I didn't know I had. If you believe in something higher, invite that into your movement. Pray while you stretch. Reflect while you walk. Let your runs, rides, or lifts be a space where you can listen and reset. Faith might look different for you, but it can be one of the strongest forms of endurance you'll ever develop.

Music is another form of faith in its own way. It's energy you can feel. The right song can pull you out of fatigue or help you push through that last rep.

I often set my alarm to a song that instantly lifts me. It's a small detail, but it changes how I wake up. During workouts, I create playlists based on what I need: confidence, peace, joy, or release. Many days, I even dance between sets. The music you choose can shape your workout, your mood, and even your mindset for the day.

I notice this the most through my kids. Music affects them instantly. If I play something upbeat, they start jumping, laughing, and singing. If I play something slow, their energy softens. There's one song that always makes me cry—a song about kids growing up and the house becoming quiet. It reminds me to soak in these moments, the noise and chaos included. But every time it comes on, my kids ask me to skip it. They can feel the sadness. That's how powerful music is. It gets into our emotions and bodies before we even realize it. Be mindful of what you listen to. Choose what uplifts and strengthens you.

The discipline you build through fitness will eventually spill into every other part of your life. The patience you develop when you're trying to build strength will show up when you're handling challenges at work or at home. The focus that helps you finish a tough workout will be the same focus that helps you navigate hard conversations, financial goals, or parenting struggles. That's why the goal here is longevity.

The longer you stay committed, the easier it becomes to see that fitness is never really about the physical. It's about consistency. It's about self-respect. It's about choosing growth when staying the same would be easier. You'll know you've reached that point when working out stops feeling like a chore and starts feeling like something you need to feel like yourself again. It becomes as natural as breathing. That's what "in it for the long haul" means. It's when you stop asking, "How long will this take?" and start saying, "This is just what I needed."

There will be days when you feel unstoppable and days when you question everything. But if you keep showing up, it all adds up. You will gain the ability to fall down, rest when needed, and rise again with more clarity than before.

Taking care of your health is one of the greatest acts of self-love you can ever commit to. When you move your body, you're not just building muscle. You're also building confidence, discipline, and faith in yourself. You're showing your family, friends and even strangers what it looks like to live with intention. You're reminding yourself that you're capable of doing hard things and that you can keep going even when life shifts and gets messy. And here's the truth: there is no finish line. There's no point where you've "arrived" and can stop. This journey keeps evolving, just like you do. Some seasons, your fitness will look like running races or lifting heavy. Other times, it'll look like walking, stretching, or taking care of your mind first. It all counts.

You've made it this far because something in you wanted more. More energy. More peace. More strength. That desire doesn't go away, it grows. And as it grows, so do you.

Your Next Move: Celebrate the fact that you finished this book by moving your body today in any way that feels good. Dance, stretch, walk, or lift. Let it be your way of saying: I've started, and I'm not stopping here.

A FEW WORDS

Where are you now? Have you fit some workouts into your schedule yet? Have you had a healthy meal that made you feel good afterward? Maybe you've slept better in the last few nights, or perhaps you've simply taken a moment to check in with yourself mentally. Are you starting to entertain the idea of falling in love with fitness? Or are you still skeptical, still unsure whether any of this will work for you? That's okay too.

Nothing has to change immediately just because you've read one book. If it does, though, and you feel that spark and take off running with it, that's incredible. But if it doesn't, it doesn't mean this wasn't worth your time. Sometimes change is planted quietly, like a seed, and it takes days, weeks, or even years before it blooms. Maybe this book will point you toward something else you need. Maybe it will help you realize what the next step is for your own journey. Or maybe you'll set it down for now, and one day, a line or an idea from these pages will pop into your mind at exactly the right moment.

From the start, I've been honest with you in that I don't have all the answers. What I've shared here are simply the things that have worked for me, the tools I've gathered over years of trial, error, setbacks, and breakthroughs. I didn't discover them all at once, and I certainly didn't master them overnight. Even now, I'm still learning what works best for me in the season of life I'm in. And life is nothing if not a series of changing seasons. Some are bright and full of momentum. Others feel dark, heavy, and exhausting. Having a foundation of caring for yourself makes the hard seasons more bearable and the good seasons even better.

Whenever I'm having a bad day, month, or even a year filled with challenge after challenge, I know I can always lean on one constant: my health. I might not be perfect, but I can choose to move my body. I can choose to fuel myself in a way that supports me. And even if I'm not doing it every single day, I know those habits are there for me to come back to, and they will catch me when I need them.

I've always said that taking care of your body inside and out is a kind of cheat code for life. I'm human. I make mistakes. I have moments when I want to quit. But the discipline of caring for my health has allowed me to show up better in every role I play, whether that be wife, mother, daughter, sister, friend, colleague, all of it. So why wouldn't you want to give yourself that gift?

Take everything one step at a time. Let yourself be a work in progress. And little by little, watch yourself fall in love with fitness.

Your Next Move: Do not just close this book. Make a plan. Pick a race, challenge, or training program that excites you. Set a start date within the next two weeks. Put your workouts on the calendar. Tell one person who will hold you to it. Then begin. Show up and repeat.

ACKNOWLEDGMENTS

ACKNOWLEDGMENTS

This book wouldn't exist without the people who poured into me along the way.

To my husband, Gavrin. Thank you for asking how it's going, swapping workout days, and making sure I continued writing even when life was busy and messy. You keep me on my A-game and push me to be the best version of myself.

To my kids, Genevieve, Gabriel & Giovanni. You have been my loudest cheerleaders, reminding me to finish this book and celebrating every small step forward. You've shown me what real strength looks like.

To my mommy, Manette. This book carries your fingerprints. You encouraged every mile, every race, every dream. You made space for me to work on it, and though you're not here physically to see it finished, your love is embedded in every word.

To my dad, Guy. Thank you for teaching me to love words from a very young age, to write with intention, to speak with clarity and to always believe in myself no matter what anyone says. Those lessons and that love live in every chapter.

To my siblings (Lamarre, Guilise, Charlotte and Andrew), extended family and my dearest friends. Your encouragement, laughter, and support kept me moving when it would have been much easier to stop. You know who you are, and I'm beyond grateful for you.

To my fitness community. Both in person and online. Thank you for your stories, your energy, and your trust. You've inspired me as much as I hope to inspire you.

And to you, the reader. Thank you for letting my story into your life. I hope these pages encourage you, challenge you, and remind you that movement can carry you through anything.

ABOUT THE AUTHOR

Florence "Flo" Gondré Brown, MA, EdM, is a runner, marathon finisher, and wellness creator passionate about helping others fall in love with taking care of their total bodies: mind, heart, and soul included. With a background in counseling and a deep understanding of how movement shapes mental health, Flo blends expertise and empathy to help others find strength in every season of life.

As a mom of three and the voice behind several fitness and mindset guides, Flo brings honesty, humor, and heart to everything she creates. Whether she's training for her next race, crafting a wellness guide, or cheering from the sidelines at her kids' games or performances, she continues to live the message she teaches: that movement is a form of self-love and that showing up for yourself is always worth it.

WORKS CITED

Blumenthal, J.A., Smith, P.J., & Hoffman, B.M. (2012). Opinion and Evidence: Is Exercise a Viable Treatment for Depression? ACSM's Health & Fitness Journal, 16(4), 14–21. https://doi.org/10.1249/01.FIT.0000416000.09526.eb

Harvard T.H. Chan School of Public Health. (2015). Many adults played sports when young, but few still play. https://www.hsph.harvard.edu/news/press-releases/poll-many-adults-played-sports-when-young-but-few-still-play/

Mandal, S. (2020). How to make your New Year's resolutions work? Social Behavior Research and Practice Open Journal, 4(2), 28–29. https://doi.org/10.17140/SBRPOJ-4-119

Matthews, G. (2007). The Impact of Commitment, Accountability, and Written Goals on Goal Achievement. Dominican University of California, Psychology Faculty Conference Presentations. https://scholar.dominican.edu/psychology-faculty-conference-presentations/3

Murtagh, E.M., Murphy, M.H., & Boone-Heinonen, J. (2010). Walking: the first steps in cardiovascular disease prevention. Current Opinion in Cardiology, 25(5), 490–496. https://doi.org/10.1097/HCO.0b013e32833ce972

Today@USC. (2023). Can student-athletes maintain their fitness for life? https://today.usc.edu/can-student-athletes-maintain-their-fitness-for-life/

Verywell Mind. (2023). What is a self-fulfilling prophecy? https://www.verywellmind.com/what-is-a-self-fulfilling-prophecy-6740420

World Health Organization. (2023). Depression fact sheet. https://www.who.int/news-room/fact-sheets/detail/depression

WORKS CITED

Psychology Today. (2016). Study: If you believe in exercise, it'll make you feel good. https://www.psychologytoday.com/us/blog/the-athletes-way/201608/study-if-you-believe-in-exercise-itll-make-you-feel-good